Sex Position Guidebook

The ultimate guide with pictures about Kama sutra, tantric sex and advanced sex techniques to make your partner scream

by

Scarlett Hunter

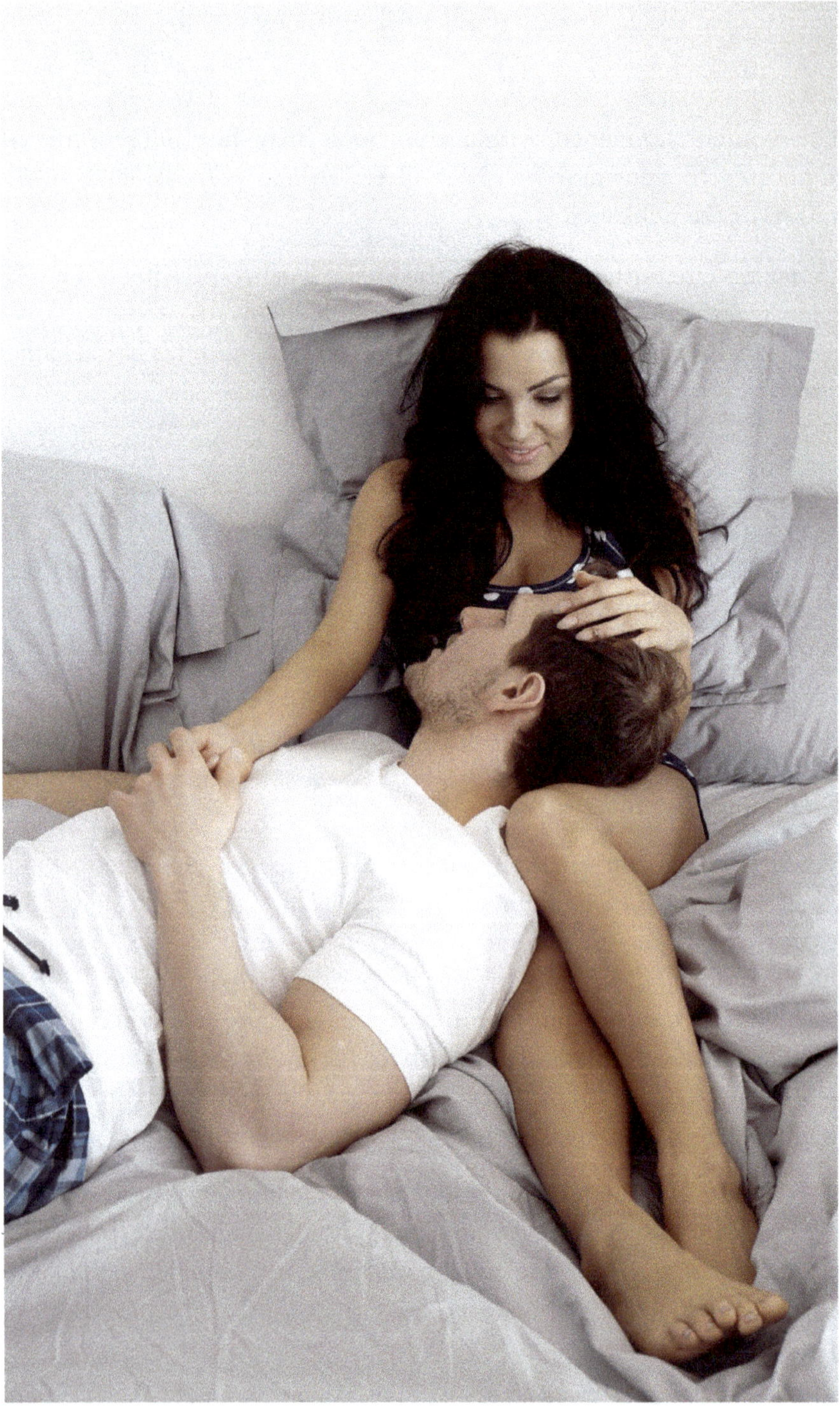

Table of Contents

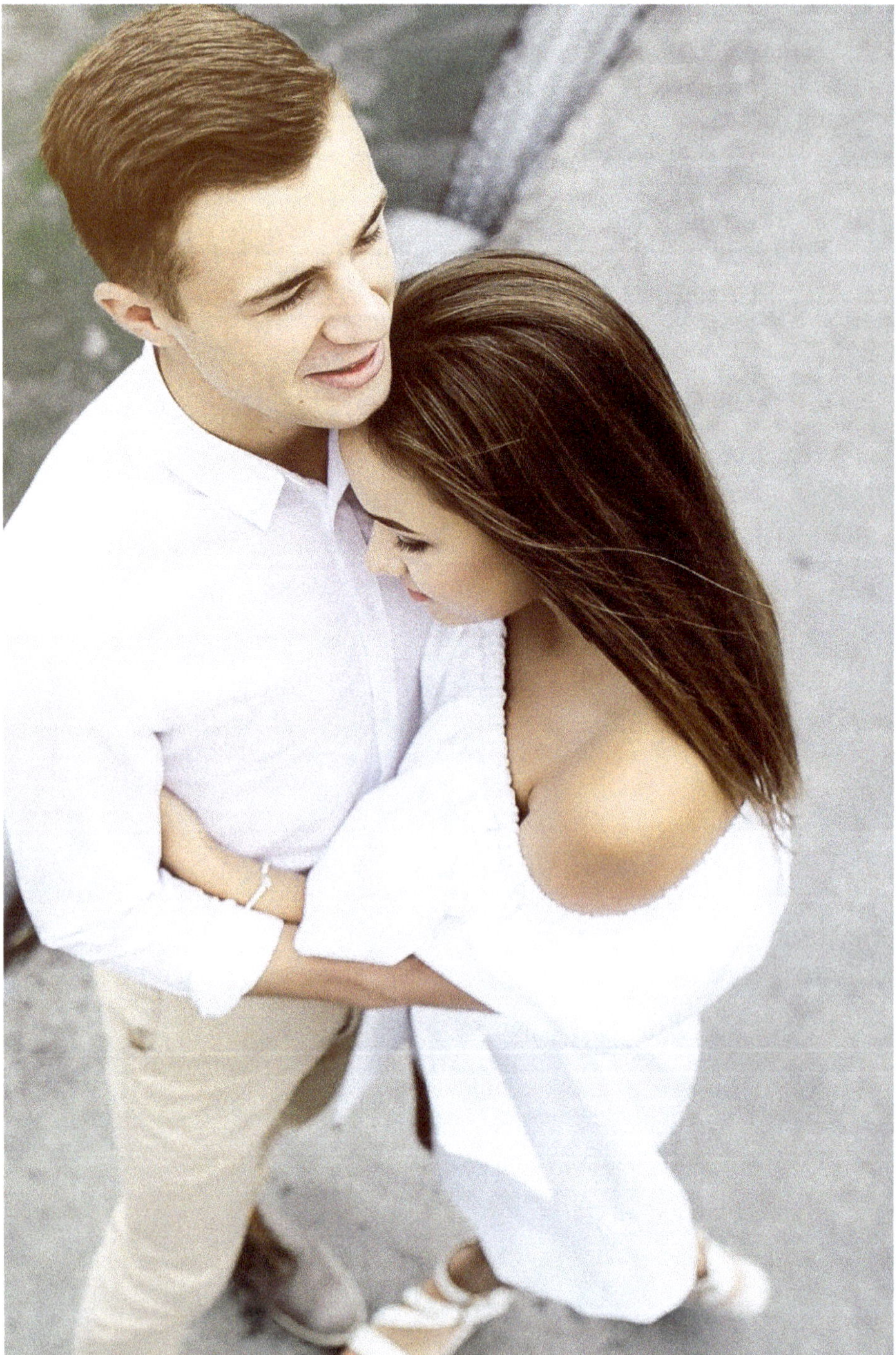

Introduction

Congratulations on purchasing *Sex Position Guidebook*, and thank you for doing so. The following chapters will discuss the essential elements of having tantric sex and the best ways that you and your lover can improve your sex life for a much happier time.

There are plenty of books on this subject on the market, thanks again for choosing this one! Every effort was made to ensure it is full of as much useful information as possible. Please enjoy!

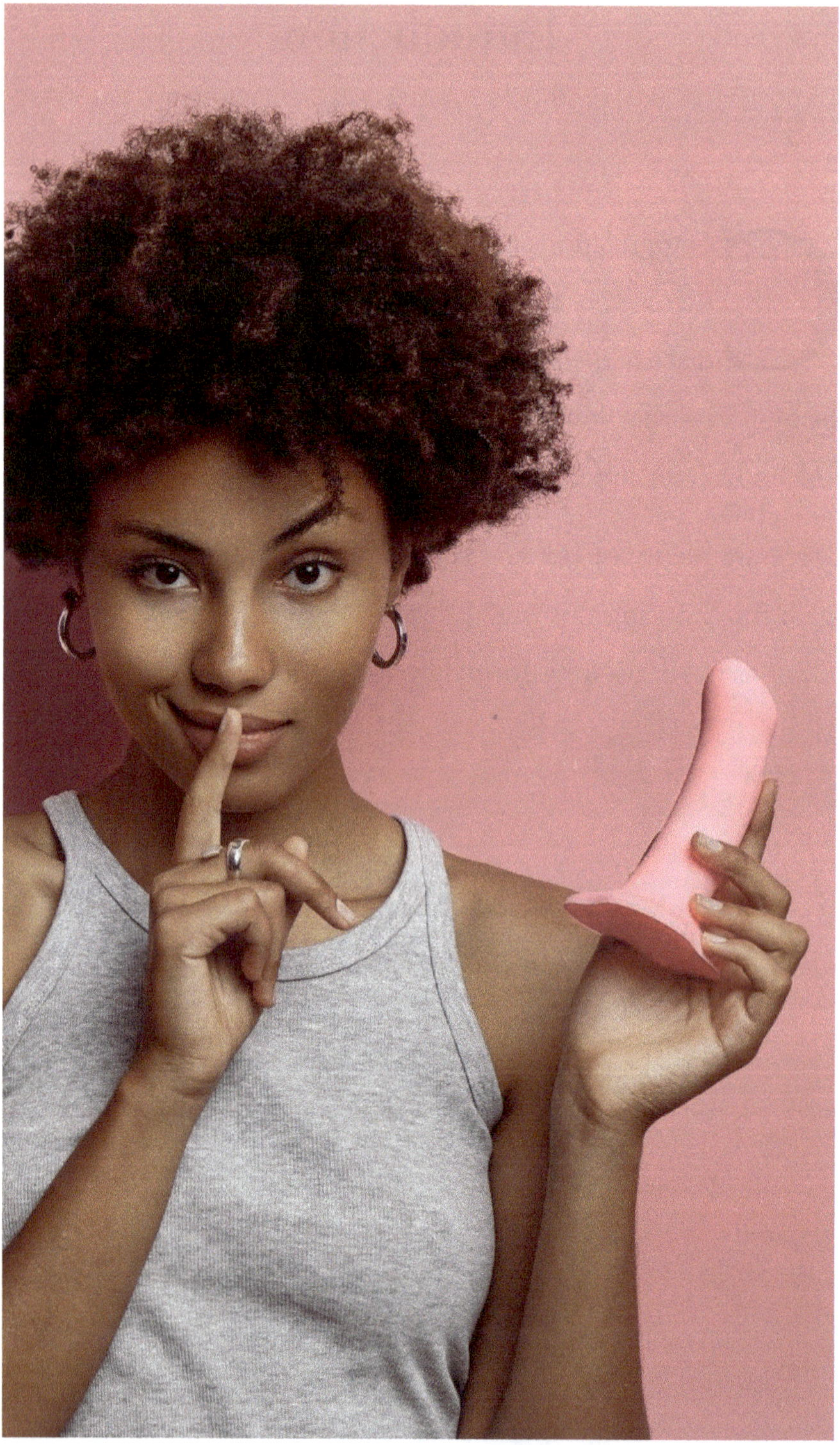

Chapter 1:
Brief History of Tantra

Tantra is not a religion, albeit Tantric symbology and practices have risen from the beginning of time in all religions and societies. Portrayals of the sacrosanct association of the manly and female standards and the non-duality of this "holy internal marriage" can be found as far back as 2000 BC in the Indus Valley development and the old Egyptian kingdom.

Tantric standards are innate in otherworldly Judaism (Kabbalah), Christianity and Sufism. Chinese Taoism is another strand of Tantra.

Tantra most clearly developed in India, somewhere in the range of 300 and 400 CE, when the main Hindu and Buddhist Tantric writings were recorded as graceful illustrations indicating unity and Divine love. These first works were intentionally dark with the goal that no one but starts could get them.

Prior to that time, Tantric lessons were firmly watched and transmitted orally from ace to teach simply after extensive stretches of planning and purification.

Tantra arrived at its peak in the eleventh and twelfth hundreds of years, when it was rehearsed generally and transparently in India. Tantra invalidated the predominant idea that freedom could be achieved uniquely through thorough austerity and by the renunciation of the world.

Tantrikas (tantric yogis) accepted that human experience emerges the mixed up thought of partition. It pushed festivity of the exotic and, through so doing greatness of the physical.

Tantra has been and still is polished in three principal shapes: the religious convention, the householder custom and by meandering yogis. Though Hinduism had numerous guidelines and laws, including severe divisions of the station, Tantra was absolutely non-denominational and could be polished by anybody, even inside everyday life.

In this manner, reflections on weaving, for instance, could be drilled by weavers, as they thought about the interlaced and undifferentiated nature of presence, while interventions on eating, drinking and lovemaking could be rehearsed by lords and rulers.

With the intrusion of India in the thirteenth century came across the board butcher of Tantrics and annihilation of their original copies. Tantra went underground, where it has transcendently stayed since.

Tantric Buddhism was strikingly safeguarded in the religious communities of Tibet. After the Chinese attack of Tibet, when priests and nuns were killed and original copies wrecked, the individuals who got away have discovered approaches to delicately disperse this learning all the more broadly.

It is standard to separate Tantric ways into two segments. Those where the individual professional works with his/her own sexual vitality, for the most part inside, are classified "right-gave" ways or "white Tantra." At that point, there are Tantric methodologies that do include direct sexual contact between affection accomplices, and these are designated "left-gave" Tantra or "red Tantra." These terms, be that as it may, are themselves part of a progressively present-day arrangement of classification.

In the west, today, conventional Tantric practices can be found inside the Tibetan Buddhist custom and using the Kundalini and Kriya yoga schools, which are all right-gave ways.

There is additionally the Taoist custom, which has just somewhat been modified, and this is a left-gave way. Daniel Odier was started by Lalita Devi in the Himalayas, in the genealogy of Kasmimir Shaivism.

The primary practices that he instructs are sitting contemplation, the "tandava," a type of extremely unpretentious free development, where experts contact an ever-increasing number of refined conditions of the "divine tremoring" a reverberation with the pith of life, and Kashmiri vitality knead.

Generally, Tantric experts did not promote themselves, and this is, for the most part, still obvious today. Many exist, especially in India, in the west as well, however, you will not discover such a large number of Tantric bosses by means of the web.

The birthplace of the tantric customs is a puzzler, to a great extent because of the scarcity of recorded proof in India from the period when it appears that they originally developed during the Gupta line (320–550 C.E.). This scarcity of proof has prompted a lot of unbridled theory with respect to the birthplace of these customs. There is no hard proof for the presence of tantric conventions before the mid-first thousand years C.E.

While obviously a few parts of the tantric customs, for example, trademark practices or iconography, extensively originate before the chronicled development of these conventions, the different endeavors to date Tantrism preceding the primary thousand years C.E. depend on extremely feeble proof.

The tantras themselves, just as related sacred writings (*āgama, saṃhitā*, and so on), are comprehended by their separate conventions to be uncovered works, at first educated by gods. In the *Śaiva* convention, sacred texts are accepted to have begun in lessons given by *Śiva* to his wife, *Devī*; these lessons were then later passed on to human sages, for example, *Matsendranāth*.

The *Śākta* and *Vaiṣṇava* tantric customs, then again, hold the Goddess and *Viṣṇu*, individually, to be the first divine educator. Some Buddhist tantric customs guarantee that their sacred writings were instructed by enormous ageless buddhas and afterward uncovered to adepts.

These legends, while guaranteeing that sacred writings begin in an immortal awesome articulation, in any case, point to their disclosure as being ruminated by extraordinary acknowledged adepts (*mahāsiddhas*) who lived during the early medieval period, around the seventh through thirteenth hundreds of years, pretty much when most tantric sacred texts really became known.

To the degree that tantric sacred texts examine their starting points, these divulgences will, in general, be legendary as opposed to authentic. Regarding these legends as history is normally methodologically unsound.

For instance, various Buddhist tantras, following the literary model of the Buddhist sūtra kind, start with an opening section (*nidāna*) that shows the conditions where the sacred text was educated. Various tantras guarantee that they were, similar to the sūtras, at first instructed by *Śākyamuni* Buddha.

Notwithstanding these starting point claims, in any case, there is positively no proof that any of the Buddhist tantras began when the Buddha lived, around the fifth century B.C.E. These sections speak to endeavors to real these functions as stirred discourse (*buddhavacana*) and cannot be taken as authentic proof.

While endeavors to root parts of tantric conventions in the far off past are theoretical, best-case scenario, there is no uncertainty that these customs, as they rose, were intensely subject to prior Indian conventions of idea and practice.

Perhaps the greatest effect on tantric customs was the far more seasoned Vedic convention of Hinduism. Vedic Hinduism highlighted the holy class, *Brahmins*, who had the sacrosanct obligation to remember the oral holy writing of the custom, the Vedas, and furthermore become familiar with the intricate ceremonial practices the convention supported. These ceremonies concentrated on contributions to the divine beings made into a consecrated flame, which ran from to a great extent vegan contributions made into little local (*gṛhya*) fires that householders were to keep up to the bigger "serious" (*śrauta*) customs that required creature sacrifice.

This convention created around 1500–500 B.C.E., arriving at its pinnacle directly around 500 B.C.E., only before the ascent of the renunciant customs that would challenge it. In spite of the fact that there was a strain between promoters of the Vedic convention and supporters of a portion of the tantric customs, the tantric conventions drew intensely from Vedic ceremony practice customs regardless.

This getting incorporates a discount adjustment of the key Vedic custom of flame sacrifice, *homa*, and the change of the Vedic ceremony of regal sanctification, *rājyasūya*, into the tantric ritual of inception *qua* "sanctification," *abhiṣeka.*

Indeed, even the particularly tantric routine with regards to picturing oneself as a divinity had Vedic forerunners; some Vedic customs required custom identification with the God, by means of both internal representation and external ceremonial activities.

This was a characteristic result of the decay of the Vedic śrauta sacrificial framework around the fifth through thirteenth hundreds of years. Furthermore, its decrease was joined by the parallel ascent of the tantric conventions, which grew new ceremonial frameworks that obtained intensely from Vedic forerunners.

One of the key elements prompting the rise of the tantric conventions was the ascent of the world-revoking *śramaṇa* development a thousand years sooner around the mid-first thousand years B.C.E. This development, which began inside Hinduism yet prompted the advancement of adversary conventions, to be specific Buddhism and Jainism, was portrayed by its featuring of the objective of freedom (*mokṣa*) from the cyclic presence (*saṃsāra*) as the key religious objective, just as the verbalization of unmistakable ways of training for arriving at this objective.

These incorporate, most remarkably, renunciation and plainness as a key essential for freedom. Buddhist and Hindu *śramaṇa* customs held that freedom came about because of a procedure of "enlivening" (*bodhi*) in which the expert accomplishes a unique information or gnosis (*jñāna*) that frees one from the cycle of enlivening.

The act of contemplation and yoga were viewed as key practices to build up this acknowledgment. Tantric customs acquired this suspicion, and a significant number of the pondering practices, from prior renunciant conventions.

Buddhist tantric conventions, normally, acknowledged the cosmological and philosophical structures created by before Buddhist customs, just as a significant number of their pensive practices.

Hindu tantric customs, thusly, acknowledged and further built up the modern cosmological and mental principles created by the *Sāṃkhya* school, just as the pensive practices created by its sister Yoga school. Both of these conventions encouraged the transmission of thoughts and practices created by Hindu *śramaṇa* gatherings.

The early first thousand years C.E. likewise observed another significant advancement in Hinduism, in particular, the ascent of the Bhakti reverential development.

This improvement happened around a similar time as the ascent of the tantric conventions. It was portrayed by a propensity toward monotheism, in that dedication to a solitary preeminent maker god was viewed as the way to salvation.

This inclination is antiquated in Hinduism and is extremely clear in a portion of the later Upaniṣads dating to the second 50% of the principal thousand years B.C.E. Generally early works, for example, the Bhagavad Gīta, assessed to date around 100 C.E., call for commitment to God as the preeminent way to freedom.

The prominence and touchy development of reverential Hinduism significantly affected the tantric conventions. Dedication to God is a focal element of most Hindu tantric conventions, and the *Vaiṣṇava* Pāñcarātra custom specifically melded both Bhakti and tantric methods of training.

Given Buddhism's dismissal of the idea of a preeminent Creator God, one would expect that the Bhakti impact would be less obvious in Buddhist tantric customs. This might be the situation; however, while the impact was less, it was not nonexistent.

In the Buddhist setting, commitment is ordinarily constrained to the master, however, this is viewed as a fundamental essential for tantric practice. The need of dedication to the master is emphatically underlined in later works, for example, The Fifty Stanzas on the Guru (*Gurupañcāśikā*).

The specific time where tantric customs rose in India stays a mystery because of a deficiency of recorded proof in South Asia from the main portion of the primary thousand years C.E. Nonetheless, as we will find in the following segment beneath, the accessible proof proposes that the fifth century C.E. was the no doubt time frame in which the primary tantric customs rose, and they likely rose first with regards to the Śaiva convention of Hinduism.

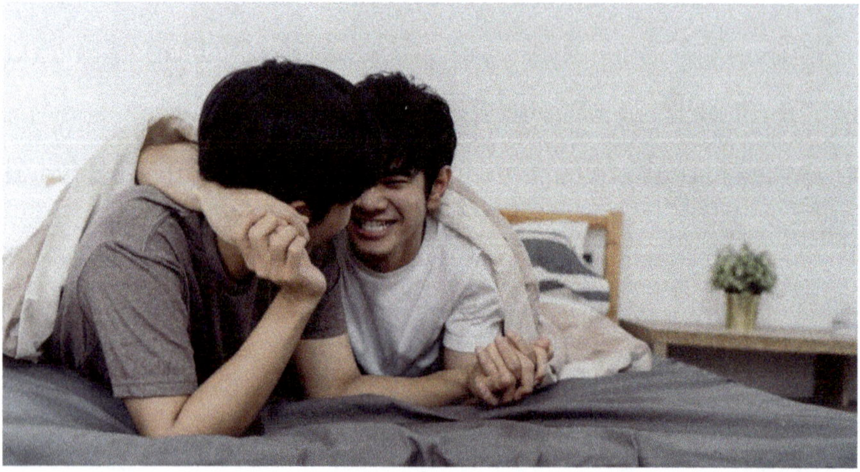

Chapter 2: Benefits of Tantric Sex

You might probably improve your sexual wellbeing through the act of tantric yoga and sex. Tantric yoga includes a few activities, including the ground-breaking blend of asana, mantra, mudra, bandha, and chakra, that lead to a solid and euphoric life.

Tantric sex is a moderate type of closeness that may build closeness and a mind-body association that regularly causes solid climaxes.

This blend of having a solid body, brain, and soul association, alongside various, amazing sexual climaxes, will have cherishing couples invigorated by expanding the emission of the pineal and pituitary organs.

Sexual Health Improves

Some cases that tantric sex has a restoring impact, improving people's sexual wellbeing. Visit climaxes, as one of the cerebrum wave reenactments, may change body science. Sorrow and stress may vanish. A lady's sexual wellbeing might be incredibly improved.

In tantric sex, the cerebrum science might be influenced by enabling the endocrine organs for more HGH, serotonin, DHEA, and testosterone. Scientific and therapeutic examinations have recommended that sex improves wellbeing radically by animating blood flow, detoxifying the body through the breath, and fortifying cardiovascular, endocrine/insusceptible, and anxious capacities.

For instance, an examination done by Wilkes University found that creation love, in any event, two times every week discharges a counteracting agent considered immunoglobulin An or IgA, which may shield the body from the ailment.

Climaxes Strengthen Immune System

Climaxes may help ease gloom and make you look and feel more youthful. Some trust it can likewise draw out your lifespan, reinforce the safe framework, and improve in general wellbeing.

In any case, increasingly broad clinical examinations are expected to affirm these outcomes.

Could sexual introduction to semen battle misery and lift temperaments in the two ladies and men? It might be that hazardous and unprotected sex may prompt despondency, while secured sex can give disposition upgrades, enthusiastic bonds, and closeness.

In this way, people may infer incredible advantages by expanding the sexual amount and sexual quality in a protected, solid, regular route through tantric sex. Tantric sex specifically centers around the advantages of delaying the sex represent more closeness and medical advantages.

Potential Benefits of Frequent Orgasms, Tantric Sex, and Women's Health

Visit climaxes may profit a lady's sexual wellbeing. Be that as it may, there is an immense difference between a customary climax and a tantric climax.

Normal climaxes last a brief length and stay confined in the sexual organs. Tantric sex climaxes hypothetically include the full-body, personality, and soul, and keep going for a considerable length of time.

As per antiquated practices, to get the advantages of a tantric climax, the shakti or vitality, and the rising kundalini must puncture each of the chakras (vortexes of vitality in the unobtrusive body) as it rises the spinal string.

It must arrive at the mind's focal sensory system and endocrine war room—the nerve center and pituitary organ, which directions the progressions that advantage our sexual wellbeing.

Aficionados of tantric sex accept that visit, amazing climaxes increment the degree of the climax hormone, oxytocin.

They additionally accept oxytocin levels and your climaxes influence your states of mind, energy, social aptitudes, and feelings, all of which may impact different parts of your day by day life.

Tantric sex depends on a way of thinking of oriental root that is more than 4 thousand years of age, utilizing sexual vitality to accomplish an association between bodies, without accomplishing a sexual relationship under the standards thought about ordinary by the Western culture.

This method depends on Tantra, identified with a sort of sexual move, which must be adjusted to the cadence of each couple or traditions, continually targeting accomplishing a glad sexual life, through the ease of constructive vitality inside every individual.

To do this sexual practice, a progression of statutes controlled by the Eastern culture must be connected, with some outside impacts that will make this a really life-changing background.

The principal reason to apply is to live at the time, attempt to stay away from a wide range of diversions, which implies that during the demonstration, both must be available with the brain and body to appreciate the demonstration to the most extreme.

At that point, you should acknowledge your accomplice as he/she is, without seeing physical or mental shortcomings, so you can take the relationship in full, and not just one must acknowledge the body of an individual, yet additionally the body itself, with any defects it may have.

A significant point in tantric sex is the planning of the earth where the connection will occur, so you should consider the air, light, scents, sustenance, and atmosphere; this will guarantee that the energies stream in an unbelievable manner between the two individuals.

In this sexual practice, individuals should do not hesitate to state what they think or need to do with their accomplice, on the grounds that there ought to be no hindrances, however a private correspondence between both.

The objective with tantric sex as in other sexual strategies will consistently be to arrive at the best delight conceivable, it is prescribed to keep eye-to-eye connection with your accomplice for additional power and genuinely staggering climaxes.

In this sort of eccentric practices, one must stay cool and know about the passionate and sensorial sensations, for example, contact, vision, smell, and hearing at each piece of your accomplice's body, this will produce another world brimming with conceivable outcomes for delight.

As per specialists, when performing tantric sex, individuals significantly improve their physical wellbeing because of the measure of calories that are lost in this training, which straightforwardly impacts the breath, the heartbeat and blood course.

A few examinations likewise demonstrate that a great many people experience serious phases of despondency, yet in addition state that couples who take part in tantric sex, have improved extensively from this with the disposal of pessimistic vitality and fascination of constructive ones. To do this training, the couple must consent to do as such, with the sole target to accomplish life-changing climaxes.

Dedicating yourself to any training must have settlements. There are numerous profits from putting time and vitality into tantric sex. Tantric sex practices can enable you to accomplish the accompanying:

1. ***Draw out delight.*** Tantric sex strategies make lovemaking—including the glimmer—keep going quite a while. This happens through ejaculatory control as well as

by figuring out how to coordinate sexual vitality anyplace in the body or into profound manifestations.

2. ***Enable ladies.*** Numerous ladies experience the ill effects of low confidence. They may have a poor self-perception or they may surrender to sex when they would truly like to say no or not tell their accomplice what they truly need. In tantric sex, ladies are treated with the regard and respect they want and merit.

3. ***Extend your conceivable outcomes for adoration.*** Tantric sex tells you the best way to develop the physical and otherworldly association with your accomplice, and support and love yourself.

4. ***Help you accomplish genuine fulfillment from sex.*** When the sex demonstration is finished, are you ever left with the inclination that you are not so much wrapped up? This is regularly because the sexual act does not go past the private parts—it doesn't contact the heart.
   In tantric sex, you can arrive at the state where each cell in your body feels supported from the spirit association you feel with your accomplice.

At the point when sex occurs with this sort of heart association, both body and psyche are nourished.

5. **Enable men.** Such a significant number of men stress over their penis size, and to what extent they last in sex. Numerous additionally do not have a clue how to submit or actually please a lady. At the point when men feel progressively enabled in sex, they become increasingly certain and open to being all the more minding in their relationship.

6. ***Ease nerves and wretchedness.*** Measurements show a huge number of people experience the ill effects of uneasiness and melancholy, including manifestations like weariness, listlessness, and resting and eating aggravations. Tantric sex gives a colossal wellspring of vitality to the body and tranquility to the mind that conquers these issues.

7. ***Influence the world decidedly.*** Your own additions cause you to create more positive and adoring vitality ostensibly, stretching out to everybody you come into contact with, modifying the vitality of the planet since everything on a mystical or otherworldly level are interrelated.

8. ***Raise sex.*** When you hoist sex to a degree of holiness, it takes on a more extravagant measurement than an insignificant physical act.

9. ***Tap into the wellspring of youth.*** For all the medical advantages referenced beforehand, rehearsing tantra can make you feel and look youthful once more.
10. ***Recuperate past enthusiastic injuries.*** Tantric sex can enable you to mend past damages from a wide range of difficult or horrendous encounters in which you felt double-crossed or abused. Instead, it encourages you to make encounters of being regarded in sex and in life as a rule.

11. ***Revive your wellbeing.*** Rehearsing tantric sex has physiological and mental impacts that keep up—and recover—wellbeing. For instance, breathing systems carry more air into the body, supporting the tissues and muscles. Research has demonstrated a connection between the impacts of unwinding, contemplation, and otherworldliness and better physical and passionate wellbeing. Individuals who are otherworldly have a lower circulatory strain, lower levels of uneasiness and sadness, progressively stable hormone levels, and better working invulnerable frameworks.

12. **Extend your association with others.** Tantric sex gives all the more significance to life and enhances your connections.

Chapter 3: Myths and Truths about Tantric Sex

The most widely recognized and most stunning misguided judgment about Tantra is that it is about sex. This distorted, decreasing, tight and false thought most likely began with smug Victorian ethics, and their sentiments of repulsiveness towards closeness, and has fanned out quickly all through the Western Hemisphere, where it has rotted into the present day.

Libertinism, released want, climax, happiness, wild sex, grimy sex, unusual positions, bashes, numerous accomplices, candles, incense, enchantment ceremonies, and even dark enchantment are what struck a chord when individuals hear the word 'Tantra.'

As a general rule, Tantra is one of the most significant profound Indian conventions, the viable part of Veda.

In Sanskrit, the word signifies "to weave" and originates from the expression "*tanoti*" signifying "to grow," and "*trayati*," signifying "freedom."

By rehearsing Tantra, utilizing your body, brain, detects, and energies, alongside Tantric strategies, your cognizance extends and rises above the confinements of your body and psyche.

Tantra doesn't exclusively utilize sexual vitality, the same number of think and decrease the framework to, yet every part of your being.

In this way, it causes you to change yourself through a profound work on, utilizing different systems and techniques, from Hatha-yoga, Kriya-yoga, Kundalini-yoga, Raja-yoga, Japa-yoga, and Bhakti-yoga, into an illuminated, completely mindful, person.

Every one of the energies in your body is stirred, your vitality channels are purified, and your chakras are thriving wonderfully through the different yogic practices.

Tantra offers plenty of strategies from which everybody can choose specific systems that fit their independence, that address specific issues they have at one point, and that guide them towards their individual blooming.

Tantra is definitely not a one-size-fits-all sort of thing. Yet rather, it offers a wide range of strategies that can be consolidated and custom-fitted to individuals' needs so they can achieve otherworldly success, wellbeing and prosperity, and a unified cognizance.

With Tantra, you will find out about the 5 "bodies" (the physical, vigorous, mental and passionate, insight, and euphoria body), the 7 fundamental chakras (Muladhara, Svadhisthana, Manipura, Anahata, Vishuddha, Ajna, and Sahasrara), the unobtrusive lively channels, nadis, etc.

We can comprehend Tantra just like the very substrate of life and the universe that underpins, makes, associates, interlinks, and unifies everything into Oneness. You and I, as individuals, are not separate however are in reality one, directly in this exact instant, as you read this line, regardless of whether we are miles separated.

One of the fundamental reasons for Tantra is to unite everything, to bring each part of your life into your cognizance. Along these lines, you become completely mindful of everything in your life, you grasp it, and live intentionally.

Generally, dull and common day by day exercises are presently made striking, fascinating, significant, fruitful, and comprehensive, as you jump into them with an extended awareness, not a missing personality.

With the assistance of different procedures and strategies from antiquated, sacrosanct Tantra messages, every one of your possibilities bloom, all your vitality channels become unblocked, every one of your energies intensify and refine.

Your 5 faculties stir, your essentialness builds, your psyche moves toward becoming laser-sharp, and your heart opens. Your view on life, the world, and the universe augments and wises up, your awareness ventures into unendingness and winds up one with the Divine Consciousness.

Different conventions separate the common from the otherworldly, matter from the soul, want for joy from profound yearning – this division will end in an inward battle and estrangement. This sets a definite way to blame, low confidence, low fearlessness, wantonness, and bad faith.

Rather, Tantra accepts the individual as one seems to be, imperfections and all, with all the common wants, the highs and lows, and unifies one's being into wholeness.

Naturally, Tantra "weaves" together with all parts of your being, and it encourages you to grow your cognizance.

The texture of life for what it is worth, brilliant, not simply high contrast, can give you complete satisfaction in all parts of your being, correct where you are, doing precisely what you cherish and need to do.

Tantra doesn't invalidate, expel or dismiss anything, the same number of societies, otherworldly ways and religions do. A normal, purported "otherworldly searcher" consistently attempts to "get someplace," "arrive at some higher spot," "go into the light," neglecting to perceive that all is light, all is awareness.

Tantra rises above impediments and unifies what is isolated. By rehearsing it, you are not "going" anyplace or "getting" someplace; however, you are uncovering yourself. You are awakening to your actual nature and the genuine idea of all things, as they truly seem to be.

With its far-reaching, shifted, and significant arrangement of strategies and methods (counting yoga stances, pranayama, mantras, mudras, mandalas, Kundalini procedures, perception systems, Ayurveda, soothsaying, and other elusive, profound, and exceptionally otherworldly rehearses) Tantra is intended to combine the common and otherworldly. It changes you into a unified, focused, entire person, as one with the universe.

Tantra is not something you practice away from the world and society. Tantra is living, it is simply the world, it IS life. It is an approach to carry on with your life without limits.

It encourages you to know about polarities, the yin and the yang you have inside and amicably adjusted them in flawless harmony. Tantra is not "This" or "That", it IS "This" and IS "That." The crude side of life, the wild of presence, the untamed, the high and low, the smoothness and disturbance, the highly contrasting, they are all pieces of life, they are altogether incorporated into the celestial.

Tantra consolidates the human side of us with the light of the awareness, in a hallowed association. Each part of our being is uncovered, uncovered and divinized. Nothing remains out.

Vitality is called Shakti, The Divine Feminine Principle, Mother Nature, Divine Mother. Cognizance is Shiva, the Divine Masculine Principle, Heavens, Spirit. Every lady encapsulates both perfect standards, and each man encapsulates both awesome standards in different extents. That is the excellence and mystery of extremity.

In Tantra, both men and ladies are venerated as consecrated and perfect, and they ought to worship each other as encapsulations of the Divine Principles.

Their bodies are not insignificant physical vehicles of the Spirit, however blessed sanctuaries that conceal a horrible, inestimable, and gigantically amazing power inside them: Kundalini Shakti.

- **The Dance among Shakti and Shiva, vitality and cognizance, makes Life**

Everything is vitality. Quantum material science expresses the equivalent. Be that as it may, Tantra realized it sometime before them every one of, approximately a large number of years prior.

Vitality and Consciousness are something very similar. We are made of vitality and awareness, which, Tantra states, are the same.

In opposition to prevalent thinking, tantric sex is not an unusual business. The fundamental objective of tantric sex is that there is none, and the main point is to associate profoundly and profoundly with your accomplice. The peak or climax itself is not the need; rather, the voyage of investigation, finding out about one another and building a more grounded, progressively personal relationship is principal.

- **It is for weirdos**

Tantric sex has more to do with your frame of mind than everything else, so a straightforward shift in believing is everything necessary.

In India, not exclusively are most ladies totally uninformed of the idea of tantric sex, but on the other hand, are concerned there are marks of disgrace appended to it. Tantric sex appears to be a fascinating, if entirely out-there, idea.

- **You should be adaptable**

The thought behind tantric sex is to intertwine the male body, psyche and soul.

This can be accomplished by controlling your breathing, while your accomplice controls his, having intercourse in specific positions, so you are up close and personal and taking a gander at one another, and invigorating each other to delay the entire sexual procedure.

- **You need heaps of time**

Tantric sex does not imply that you need to have intercourse for quite a long time. Rather, illumination and having an adoration for your accomplice that keeps going past the length of any climax is at the center of the lessons.

It is amusing that a remark Sting made more than 20 years back still has a suffering hang on the open's creative mind. He's attempted to clarify it away in different ways. At a certain point, he said that he lamented owning the expression and didn't generally feel he could discuss the subject past saying that his wife, Trudy, is his congregation.

That is a lot nearer to what the soul of tantric sex is about. It is surely got nothing to do with boasting about resilience.

It looks to not just arrive at a definitive degree of joy by conceding his and your climaxes, yet in addition to turning out to be nearer with your accomplice and seeing every others' bodies better. The tantric methodology has unquestionably more to do with your psychological methodology than with strategy. Difficult positions are not really the way to tantric sex. "Focusing on straightforward positions, which are charming to both of you, will help drag out the erection and add to raise the joy further.

- **Search for time to attempt the accompanying**

1. Breathe in a state of harmony.
2. Keep your hands two crawls from his body at first and get the vitality he is radiating. At that point, gradually trade this vitality and start contacting and animating one another.
3. Sit bare with your accomplice, leg over leg, encompassed by pads. The room ought to be dull or faintly lit with candles. Play some delicate music.
4. Look profoundly into one another's eyes. Try not to gaze, yet see him in a manner to reveal to him that he's magnificent.

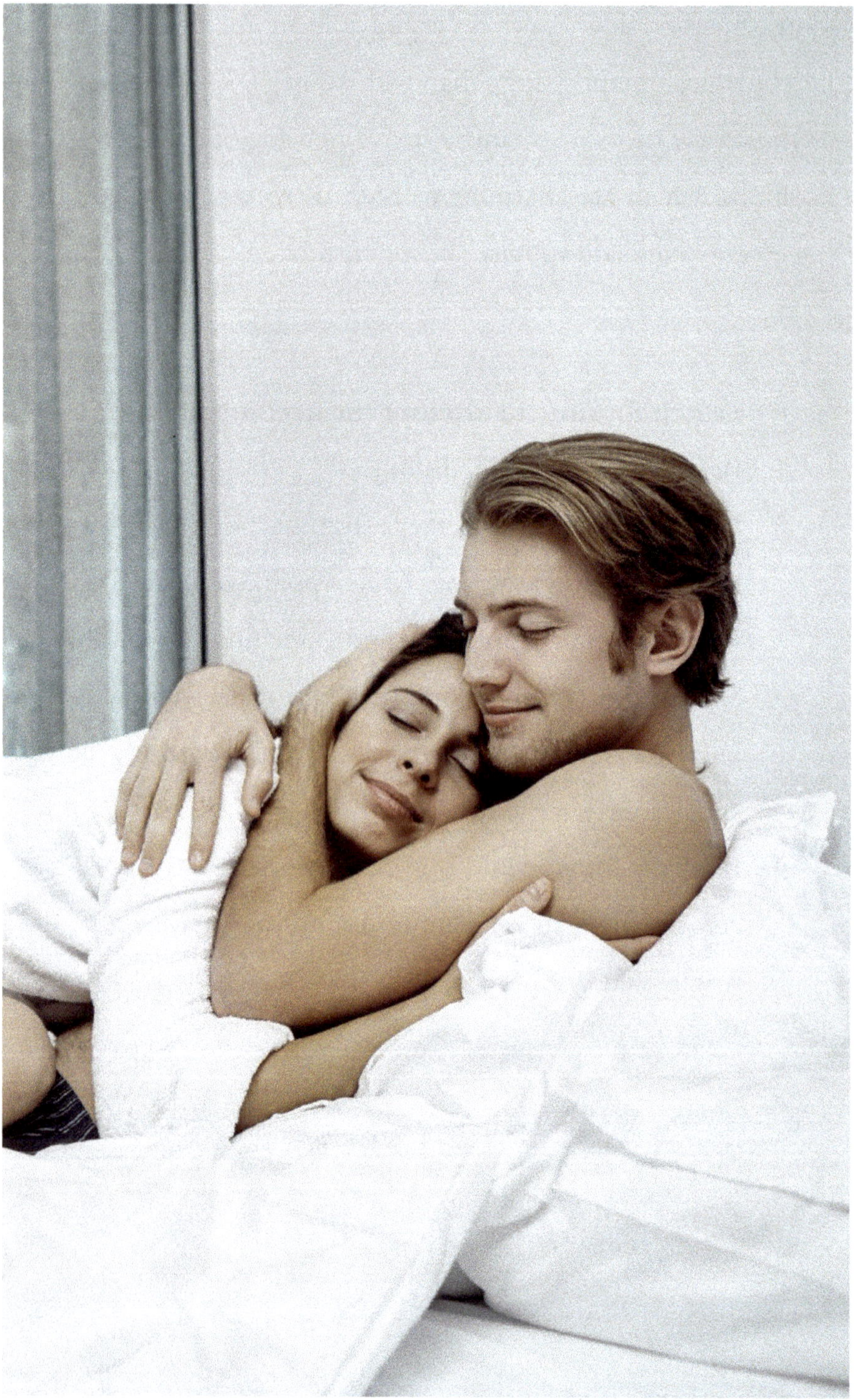

Chapter 4: Yantra

Yantra is an enchanted chart utilized in the Indian religions and reasoning for love. It is utilized to help in contemplation and for the advantages of its implied mysterious forces dependent on Tantric writings and Hindu crystal gazing. It is a sort of mandala, which is an otherworldly image speaking to the universe.

In old style Sanskrit, the word "*Yantra*," signifies "instrument," "device," or "creation." It is gotten from the root word, yam, signifying "to help" or "to continue the quintessence of an item/idea."

Yantra alludes to any sort of instrument or machine that guides a venture; however, the importance has extended to allude to religious undertakings too.

Similarly, as mantras balance the body and psyche through sound, yantras give balance outwardly. They are geometric and incorporate botanical plans. The shapes are accepted to have an amazing calming impact on the psyche, as are utilized in yogic contemplation practice. Yantras are regularly connected with a specific god and might be worn as a charm.

Among the shapes utilized in yantras are squares, triangles, circles and flower designs, however increasingly complex images might be utilized, each with significance. A lotus bloom symbolizes the chakra vitality focuses; a bindu (speck) signifies both the purpose of creation and the limitless universe; a triangle means extroversion or manliness with an upward point, and inner-directedness or womanliness with a descending point; and a swastika symbolizes karma and thriving.

The term "*Yantra*" is gotten from the Sanskrit root word "*yam*," which means supporting the embodiment of an item; and "*tra*" originates from "*trana*" or freedom from subjugation. In this way, Yantra basically implies freedom from birth and resurrection.

Yantra, Mantra, and Mandala

A Yantra is what could be compared to the Buddhist Mandala. It truly implies a 'machine' or a visual instrument that serves in contemplation.

It is a microcosm of the universe. Yantra is different from Mantra in that, Yantra is the body or type of the god, while Mantra is the psyche.

How Are They Made?

Yantras are made through the amalgamation of different geometric structures and examples that show the mind the intensity of fixation and core interest.

The drawing of a Yantra needs exactness, discipline, focus, tidiness, and accuracy. The visual structure of a Yantra actuates the correct side of the equator, which is visual and non-verbal.

Normal Yantras and Their Benefits

Sri Yantra, otherwise called Sri Chakra is the mother of all Yantras. It is the most observed Yantra in India. It speaks to Mount Meru, the enormous mountain at the focal point of the universe.

The Linga Bhairavi, as per Sadhguru, offers two Yantras, the Bhairavi Yantra and the Avighna Yantra. The Bhairavi Yantra is intended to improve the prosperity of a person. Avighna Yantra removes impediments from the life of a person.

Shakta Yantras speak to any type of the heavenly mother. These are the wellsprings of preeminent learning.

- The Astrological Yantras are utilized to bridle the energies of the nine noteworthy planets.
- The Numerical Yantras are not made out of geometrical structures, however, of numbers which fill in as charms.

- The Architectural Yantras are utilized for the ground arranging of terrains.

What Do the Various Shapes Indicate?

Each state of a Yantra transmits a quite certain, useful and agreeable vitality design that is utilized in reflection. It is a geometrical example made of a few concentric figures like squares, circles, lotuses, triangles, and focuses.

It is accepted that the concentric figures steadily become away from the middle, which signifies the procedure of macrocosmic advancement. When they bit by bit develops towards the middle, it is an image of microcosmic involution. It is a continuous development from solidarity to variety and again back to solidarity.

A human body is viewed as the absolute best and amazing of all Yantras and is viewed as an instrument for inward mindfulness.

Different Concentric Shapes

A Black point, or a Dot, or Bindu, in a Yantra, symbolizes extraordinary fixation. This point is the focal point of the Yantra and signifies solidarity.

The point ventures into a Circle or Chakra, which speaks to flawlessness and a merry inventive void.

The Triangle or Trikona in a Yantra is the image of Shakti, the ladylike vitality or the part of Creation. If the triangle focuses downwards known as Shakti Kona, it speaks to the ladylike sexual organ. If the triangle focuses upwards known as Shiva Kona, it signifies serious profound desire.

The Six Points Star or Satkona is the superimposition of the two triangles, one pointing upwards and the different downwards. This is otherwise called David's Star. This star symbolizes the association of Purusha and Prakriti or Shiva-Shakti, to shape Creation.

The Square or Bhupura is the outside furthest reaches of the Yantra. It is a symbolical portrayal of the component earth. The beginning from the Bindu to the external Square speaks to the feeling of all-inclusive development.

The Lotus or Padma in a Yantra symbolizes both immaculateness and assortment. This likewise speaks to an opportunity from various obstructions with the outside virtue.

Different Benefits

- Yantras are intended to dispose of inadequacy, unfortunate contenders, disdain, and awful impacts of planets.

- Genuine contemplation through Yantras may pull in thriving, plenitude, prosperity and good karma in all circles of life.
- It is accepted that these can bolster the expanding stream of riches.
- These Yantras have been demonstrated to successfully repulse negative energies and keep up inward amicability among the searchers.

For the One Seeking

- A Yantra works when you look at a Yantra day by day and serenade petitions to it.
- With genuine dedication, Yantras change the examples of your psyche into propensities for ideas that could get the ideal results.
- You center your goals, wants and desires in an amicable manner with the significant Mantras.
- You offer incense sticks and new blooms to it at any rate once every week upon the arrival of the god of the Yantra.

Chapter 5: Mantra

With profound practices like yoga and contemplation winding up progressively prevalent, it appears as though everybody is discussing mantras.

Be that as it may, what precisely is a mantra and how are you expected to utilize it?

In our westernized, cutting edge otherworldly rehearses, "mantra" has progressed toward becoming as standard as "goal." But the two are entirely different.

The word mantra can be stalled into two sections: "man," which means mind, and "tra," which means transport or vehicle. As such, a mantra is an instrument of the psyche—a ground-breaking sound or vibration that you can use to enter a secret government of reflection.

Like a seed planted with the goal of blooming into a beautiful lasting, a mantra can be thought of as a seed for invigorating an aim.

Much similarly you plant a blossom seed, you plant mantras in the ripe soil of training. You support them and after some time they bear the product of your aim.

Yoga and Mantra

In numerous yoga studios in the West, class starts with the teacher sharing a subject for the session. The person may welcome the understudies to set an expectation for their training and may offer recommendations for mantras to use during class.

Mantras like "I am solid," "I am engaged," or "I let proceed to give up" can enable the specialist to keep up an association with the state they wish to develop during their time on the tangle.

This mantra is utilized in quiet reiteration during development to help keep the mind centered. It has been said that in yoga, Asanas are stances of the body and mantras are stances of the brain. Mantras, when utilized in this design, are progressively similar to confirmations and help to keep you associated with a specific perspective.

Sanskrit and Mantra

Getting to the old foundation, all things considered, mantra, at its center, is the premise of every single religious custom, sacred texts, and petitions.

At the point when deliberately picked and utilized quietly, mantras are said to be able to help adjust your intuitive driving forces, propensities, and burdens. Mantras, when spoken or recited, direct the mending intensity of Prana (life power vitality) and, in conventional Vedic practices, can be utilized to empower and get to otherworldly conditions of cognizance.

Mantra as a profound practice, ought to be done all the time for a while for its ideal impacts to occur. Toward the day's end, the mantra is intended to take you back to effortlessness. We live in such an unpredictable world that it is anything but difficult to lose all sense of direction in every one of the subtleties.

Mantras can enable you to hover back to the oversimplified way to deal with life and spotlight on those things that motivate you and really satisfy you.

Reflection and Mantra

At the Chopra Center, where Primordial Sound Meditation is the favored reflection method, understudies are given a customized mantra, their Bija, which is the sound vibration the Universe was setting aside a few minutes of their introduction to the world.

This mantra is rehashed quietly again and again during the reflection practice to help the understudy in rising above the action of the psyche.

The mantra is quiet and has no significance with the goal that the mind is not centered around a specific quality or result.

It is just a vehicle that causes you to access uplifted degrees of mindfulness.

Mindfulness, in this unique circumstance, alludes to the capacity to focus on the decisions you make in your regular daily existence, and perceive when something is not working so you can transform it.

Numerous individuals face a great deal of pressure every day.

You wake up, cook breakfast, feed the children, get them to class, get down to business, drink espresso for lunch, and consume the day. Before the part of the bargain, prepared to crash. At that point, you rehash the cycle the following day.

Building up a day by day contemplation practice causes you to develop an increasingly present, quiet, and adjusted lifestyle, which swells out into each other part of your life. Mantras can help take you back to that current situation with the psyche.

You've most likely heard the word mantra previously. Be that as it may, what you can be sure of is this is an otherworldly practice and it is as old as it is significant.

We will investigate what mantras are, the different ways they can be utilized, and best of all — how you can give them something to do in your very own life for mind-blowing mending, strengthening, and change.

All in all, what is a mantra? Basically, it is a word, sound, syllable, or expression that has an incredible vibration reverberation.

They are utilized in reflection, yoga, and in the otherworldly practices of Buddhism, Hinduism, and Jainism.

You can utilize a mantra to think your vitality, open your chakras, and build up your mystic mindfulness. Otherworldly expresses, when opened, can raise your awareness. This training is so convincing and powerful. You have no clue where it could take you.

Individual mantra?

An individual mantra is an explanation that spurs and motivates you to be your best self.

With an individual mantra, you confirm how you need to carry on with your life. Also, it can help propel you to finish your objectives, both actually and expertly.

What Is Mantra Healing?

It has been demonstrated that reciting, music, and mantras strongly affect our cerebrum.

Mantras are fiery sound equations that moderate us down and permit us to see everything unmistakably. They give us a point of view.

Reciting quiets, the body and actuates various normal substantial capacities and procedures. It can likewise help in mending the psyche and body from addictions, such as smoking or liquor. In addition, reciting can reinforce the resistant framework.

Reciting can lower pulse, lessen feelings of anxiety, increment hormone level execution, and abatement nervousness and gloom.

Who might have imagined that this straightforward practice could have such control?

Yoga and Om Shanti

Om Shanti is maybe one of the most notable and open mantras utilized today. If you've at any point gone to a yoga class, odds are you've heard it.

All in all, what does Om Shanti mean? Indeed, there is a very immediate interpretation of Om Shanti. That is because Om is not to such an extent as a word as it is a sound, an inclination, and a lively reverberation.

Om is said to be the sound of the universe. This single syllable incorporates the cycle of death and resurrection. Reciting the word Om carries you into an enthusiastic arrangement with the universe.

Anyway, shouldn't something be said about Shanti? Shanti is a Sanskrit word that signifies, "Harmony." Together, the Om Shanti importance is intended to pass on: Universal Peace. It is regularly utilized as a welcome in yoga as a method for recognizing a kindred expert and wishing them harmony.

The absolute first mantras were utilized by Hindus in Quite a while more than 3,000 years prior. A few hundred years after the fact, after Buddhism started to prosper, mantras started to be joined into their otherworldly practice as well. Buddhist mantras depend on the heavenly lessons of the Buddha and the bodhisattvas. Here are three conventional Buddhist mantras you probably will not have known about previously:

"Om Mani Padme Hum"

This mantra is utilized in Tibetan Buddhism. That is to say, "I currently conjure the Universal sound, the gem, the objective of Enlightenment, love, and sympathy, Lotus shrewdness, and an unadulterated unified solidarity of insight with training." This is a routine with regards to empathy. It is utilized to look for and spread compassion for oneself as well as other people.

"Om Muni Mahamuni Shakyamuniye Svaha"

This signifies, "I summon the Universal sound, Buddha nature and the shrewd one, insightful one of the Shakyans, hail to thee!"

Likewise called the Shakyamuni Mantra, this mantra is intended to energize the improvement of what Buddhists call, Buddha nature, or the looking for of Enlightenment.

"Om Vasudhare Svaha"

Additionally, called the Buddhist cash mantra, it is utilized as a supplication to the bodhisattva of earth and wealth, Vasudhara. In Buddhism, Vasudhara is believed to be the exemplification of the female soul and is the partner to the Hindu goddess, Lakshmi. Reflection mantras are an amazing method to build your care during contemplation.

They serve a point of convergence for your consideration, a similar way you may utilize a light, a photograph, or a statue. There are many contemplation mantras you can access for nothing. The best part? They go about as a type of guided contemplation to enable you to remain grounded and present.

Here is a couple to kick you off:

- "Ham-Sah." Or, "I am that." This aide advises us that we are onlookers and along these lines separate from our human encounters and enduring.
- "Aham Prema." Or, "I am Divine Love."
- "Om Shanti, Shanti, Shanti." Or, "Genuine feelings of serenity, body, and discourse."

- "Om Tat Sat." Or, "All that is."

By what means can a mantra best be utilized?

Anyway, how would you utilize a reflection mantra? When you've chosen one, you'd like to attempt, locate a peaceful spot to start your contemplation practice.

When you are prepared, set the goal for your reflection. This is the place your chosen mantra will truly sparkle. Regardless of whether you'd like to ruminate for better wellbeing, more stillness, or only for a snapshot of harmony, set that aim before you start.

When you are prepared, start your mantra. You can say it so anyone can hear or in your mind.

Keep in mind; it is anything but a race. You can say it the same number of or as multiple times as you'd like. Perhaps you have a specific number as a primary concern. Perhaps not. Essentially rehash your mantra gradually and with a goal.

Consider what your picked mantra implies. Harp on the individual words. Let the reverberation and vibration of every syllable ring.

This type of reflective practice is a ground-breaking one. Regardless of whether you've never attempted it, you will undoubtedly encounter transformative outcomes. Try it out.

Presently, in light of the fact that mantras are a 3,000-year-old profound practice doesn't mean they aren't similarly as viable today as they were in those days!

Mantras have changed throughout the years to oblige our cutting edge frames of mind and recognitions.

A mantra shouldn't be articulated in Sanskrit to hold control. A mantra simply should be something that impacts you on a significant and individual level.

Mantras are frequently utilized in contemplation as an approach to remain engaged and focused. Be that as it may, you can utilize mantras from multiple points of view.

Print one out to set up on your divider. Record one on the network board at work. Slip a post-it mantra into your companion's handbag for an additional portion of motivation.

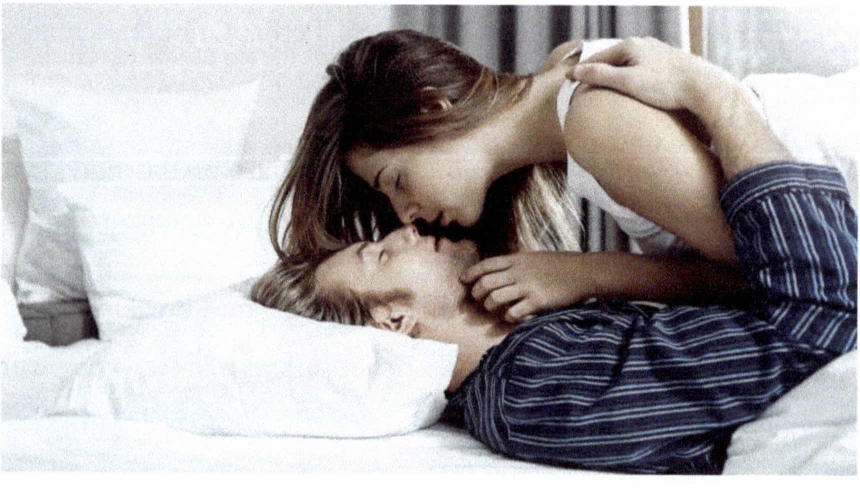

Chapter 6: Basics of Tantric Sex

Albeit frequently synonymous with sex, tantra is extremely about association — regardless of whether that is with yourself or among you and an accomplice.

All things considered, the word itself —got from the old Sanskrit— signifies "web" or "to weave vitality." by and by, tantra is about edification: to rise above both the sexual and otherworldly planes by taking part in profoundly thoughtful, unconstrained, and cozy sex.

It is tied in with becoming more acquainted with your body, and like yoga, tantra is about physical and profound mindfulness.

When you learn and practice tantra, you become more tuned in to your body, what gives it joy, and how it feels delighted. This enables you to give better consideration to your body's needs and needs and ensure they are satisfied.

Also, the energies you channel during tantric sex stream all through your body and can intensify your climax.

What's more, if you have an accomplice, becoming more acquainted with their body, as well, tantra is not just centered around arriving at a higher perspective body cognizance. It can likewise be tied in with making a more profound, progressively agreeable bond with your accomplice.

When you practice tantra, you and your accomplice figure out how to be physically mindful and profoundly present, encouraging each other vitality that keeps on developing admirably after you've completed the process of engaging in sexual relations.

Tantra additionally permits you both to investigate and extend all parts of your characters, with the goal that you start to really know the other individual all around.

Keen on rehearsing tantra, however, do not have the foggiest idea of how to approach this discussion with your accomplice? Attempt the accompanying tips:

- Give an instructor a chance to lead the way. If your accomplice is available to tantra, search out an instructor who can direct you both as you become familiar with the training.

- Tune in to what they need to state. Your accomplice may give you an eager yes or a hard no. Or then again they might be someplace in the center. Regardless of their reaction, tune in to and regard what they need to state.

- Do whatever it takes not to overpower you cooperate with data. Rather, disclose to them what you appreciate about your sex life and how you could upgrade the experience.

Setting up the Mind

Tantra is a profound practice, which means your mind becomes possibly the most important factor as much as your body.

When you practice tantra, you are interfacing your body, brain, and soul. An unmistakable attitude and ability to step out of your customary range of familiarity are imperative to joining those pieces of yourself.

A few people find that going through 5 to 20 minutes in contemplation can help set up your brain for tantra practice, as it enables you to go internal and inspect your musings.

Attempt this

Extend for a couple of minutes. As you extend every appendage, clear your psyche of any negative contemplations that are burdening you. The more you unload, the lighter you will turn into.

Go through at any rate 45 minutes every day journaling. Work through the considerations that might obstruct your profound development by keeping in touch with them down.

Concentrate on relaxing. Take 10 to 35 minutes to inhale tenderly right down into your stomach and lower back, and connect with what's happening in your psyche — regardless of whether it is pressure or satisfying your wants.

Step by step instructions to set up your space

- Tantra is a comprehensive practice. It is not about sex or climax— it is about the adventure to arrive. Your condition directly affects your outlook and your capacity to unwind and appreciate that venture.

- Fill the space with your preferred aroma. Light a scented flame, diffuse a basic oil, consume incense sticks, or hang blooms. Pick a smell that makes you feel sexy, yet is not overpowering.

- Set the disposition with candles or tinted lights. Candlelight will add sentiment to the space, while delicate red bulbs will give the territory an erotic touch.

- Mollify your space. Set out a silk toss cover and a couple of extravagant pads.

- Ensure your space is at an agreeable temperature. If it is chilly, turn on the warmth an hour prior to your training with the goal that your room is comfortable and warm. If it is hot, turn broadcasting live conditioner, however, set it to the high 70's, with the goal that the space is cool, yet not nippy.

- Make a sentimental or sexual vibe. Playing some music that you can move to, either independent from anyone else or with an accomplice.

If you are separated from everyone else

There are numerous ways you can execute tantric standards when only you are.

Be that as it may, recollect, the end game is not generally masturbation — you can work up to performance play or chose not to go there by any means.

- **Self-knead**

Make your self-knead a full-body understanding. Get your preferred oil or salve and pour it all over your skin. As you rub your oil or moisturizer in, invest energy rubbing your gut, crotch, internal thighs, arms, neck, and chest.

- **Contemplation**

Contemplation is an incredible method to free yourself of all that is keeping you down. Yet, rather than giving the vitality a chance to stream out of you, ground yourself.

As you ruminate, let your vitality stream descending into the earth. Allow that to vitality fabricate and spread all through your body, invigorating you.

- **Masturbation**

Solo play doesn't generally need to be tied in with accomplishing climax. Rather, set aside the effort to truly investigate your private parts, and what gives them —and you— delight. Contact yourself in new ways. Hinder your strokes. Mollify the manner in which you play with yourself.

Keep in mind to

- Enable yourself to encounter a full scope of feelings. This will empower you to completely take advantage of your vitality and power.

- Be available with your sensations. Rather than allowing you to mind meander, focus on everything your body is feeling.

- Set an aim for your training. Recognize what you need to escape your tantra session, regardless of whether it is to have a superior climax or to feel increasingly great in your skin.

- Inhale profoundly and gradually. Regardless of whether you are thinking or stroking off, enable your breath to interface with and send shivers down your body.

Executing with an accomplice

Keep in mind, tantra reaches out past sex — you can work up to that or decide not to go there by any stretch of the imagination.

You and your accomplice can actualize tantric standards into different practices that can develop the occasion.

- **Foreplay**

Foreplay can be anything you need it to be — oral, a back rub, scrubbing down together. Be that as it may, whatever you do, ensure you and your accomplice are completely present.

Sit before your accomplice. Investigate each other's eyes. Begin to move your bodies marginally as you relax.

Following five minutes, begin to contact each other exotically, alternating rubbing each other's arms, legs, neck, and different parts. After an additional five minutes, start to kiss — and just kiss. Concentrate on each physical sensation you are feeling at the time.

- **Sex (is discretionary!)**

You can develop to sex—or not! Tantra is more about association than all else. If you engage in sexual relations, go gradually.

What's more, do not be reluctant to be imaginative! Attempt new positions, contact each other in new ways, and investigate uncovered wants.

Be that as it may, the majority of all, drench yourself completely in the experience, giving the pressure work as you a chance to invest energy in one exotic practice before proceeding onward to the following.

- **Laying together**

Laying with your accomplice enables you to trade and weave energies, sustaining a more profound association. To do this, consider a spooning position.

The accomplice in the back will send vitality (supplier), while the accomplice in front ingests it (collector).

Cuddle near one another, with your heart and stomachs adjusted. The supplier ought to have their arms folded over the collector, with their hand over the recipient's heart.

The beneficiary should lay their hand on top. Lay still for a couple of minutes, at that point, start blending your breath and let the vitality stream unreservedly between you.

Keep in mind to

- Synchronize your relaxing. You can have a go at breathing in and breathing out together or breathing in as your accomplice breathes out.

- Allow the force construct. Look into one another's eyes without squinting for whatever length of time that conceivable.

- Set an aim for your training. Regardless of whether it is to have better sex or to reinforce your relationship, you and your accomplice ought to go into the session, realizing what you both look for from it.

- Tell your accomplice what you like. When they contact and play with you, get out what you are getting a charge out of and request that they proceed. Have your accomplice do likewise.

General Advice

Tantra is not one-size-fits-all. There are a couple of things you can do to upgrade your training to make it a wonderful — and one of a kind — experience:

- Connect the majority of your faculties. Light some scented candles. Play some delicate, arousing music. Contact yourself or your accomplice gradually.
  Gaze into one another's eyes. Appreciate the flavor of your accomplice's kisses. Connecting the majority of your faculties during your tantra practice will enable you to feel each pleasurable sensation all the more completely.

- Focus on your breath. Profound breathing is a crucial piece of tantra. By concentrating on your breath, you enable yourself to be available at the time and submerge yourself in the experience.

- Investigation. Wrinkle and BDSM, for instance, frequently fuse tantric standards. In this way, when you practice tantra, you do not need to adhere to custom. Think outside about the case — and if that implies utilizing a crate, play around with it.

- Go moderate. A significant piece of tantra is figuring out how to feel and experience everything all the more profoundly.
  What's more, the best approach to do that is to go moderate. Try not to surge tantra — rather, loosen up your psyche and appreciate each second of the training.

- Being exposed is discretionary. You can begin dressed and remain dressed or expel every last bit of texture. The key is to do whatever makes you feel good. Regardless of whether that implies being bare or not is up to you.

- Investigate the majority of your or your accomplice's body. Stroke your hands gradually over your or your accomplice's body. Give them a chance to utilize their tongue to investigate your mouth while you kiss. On the other hand, tenderly coast their lips here and there your chest. Do likewise to them.

- You do not need to go full tantra. You can add components into what you are as of now doing in the room — either independent from anyone else or with your accomplice. That could mean consolidating contemplation into foreplay or concentrating more on profound breathing during an independent session.

The most effective method to synchronize your breath

Your breath is fundamental to any tantric practice. Breathing enables you to free your psyche, associate with your body, and feel each sensation all the more completely.

When you practice any of these procedures, make sure to consistently sit upright and in an agreeable position.

The invigorating breath

This strategy can help raise vitality and increment mindfulness.

To do this:

- Breathe in and breathe out rapidly through your nose, keeping your mouth shut.
- Close your eyes and relax your tummy.
- Inhale regularly after the cycle closes, at that point, attempt again for 20 seconds, expanding by five seconds until you arrive at one entire moment.

- Attempt three in-and-out breaths every second for 15 seconds.

This procedure can enable you to discharge strain and loosen up your body. You can attempt this system while sitting opposite your accomplice, synchronizing your breath.

To do this:

- Hold your breath for a check of seven.
- Breathe out through your mouth, at that point, close your mouth.
- Breathe out through your mouth totally to a check of eight.
- Rehash the cycle three additional occasions for a sum of four breaths.

The tallying breath

Breathe in unobtrusively through your nose to a psychological check of four. This is another type of reflection that enables you to clear your brain, locate your inside, and associate with your body.

To do this:

- Give your breath a chance to stream normally.
- Close your eyes and take a couple of full breaths.

- Breathe in, at that point, check "one" to yourself as you breathe out.
- On the following breath out, check "two." Work your way up to "five."
- Rehash the cycle, beginning at "one" and closure on "five."
- Try not to go past "five," generally your brain and consideration will start to meander.
- Take a stab at checking your breath for 10 minutes.

The most effective method to get into position

Any position can be a tantric position, as tantra is about the association and not specific developments. Be that as it may, as you start your adventure into tantric standards, you might need to begin with a portion of the nuts and bolts.

Lotus

To do this with an accomplice:

- Have your accomplice sit with folded legs.
- Sit on your accomplice's upper thighs and cross your lower legs despite their good faith.
- Take in a state of harmony and gaze into one another's eyes.

To do this without anyone else's input:

- Sit leg over the leg with your back straight.
- Spot your palms on your knees.
- Start to inhale gradually and profoundly.

Hand on heart

To do this with an accomplice:

- Sit with folded legs, confronting your accomplice.
- Spot your correct hand on their heart. Have them place their correct hand on yours.
- Close your eyes, and tune into their heart's physical cadence. At that point, center around the feeling and vitality.
- Give the association a chance to work between your accomplice's heart and your hand, and the other way around.

To do this without anyone else:

- Sit leg over the leg with your back straight.
- Spot your correct hand on your heart.
- Close your eyes, and tune into its physical cadence. At that point, center around the feeling and vitality.

- Give the association a chance to work between your heart and your hand.

The casual curve

To do this with an accomplice:

- Have your accomplice sit upstanding on the bed or floor with their legs straight.
- Sit on your knees on accomplice's lap.
- Whenever agreeable, start to curve your back gradually.
- Rest your head between your accomplice's legs, at that point, seize their lower legs or feet.

To do this independent from anyone else:

- Sit on your knees on the bed or floor.
- Whenever agreeable, start to curve your back gradually.
- Lay your head on the bed or floor, at that point, stretch out your arms about your head.
- Have your palms confronting descending. Whenever prepared, utilize one hand to investigate your body.

As you become progressively versed in tantra, you will have the option to investigate and join more methods into your training, for example,

Hallowed spot rub

To do this, gradually and delicately rub your accomplice's prostate organ or the upper mass of their vagina — also called the G-spot. Give the warmth and vitality a chance to assemble, enabling your accomplice to discharge repressed out of this world closer to the peak.

Climax control

To do this, carry yourself to the edge of a climax, at that point, drawback just before you peak. Let the shivering, orgasmic sensations fill your body, at that point, start once more.

Do not simply do this one time, however — rehash the cycle again and again so you can arrive at an exceptional, unstable, full-body climax.

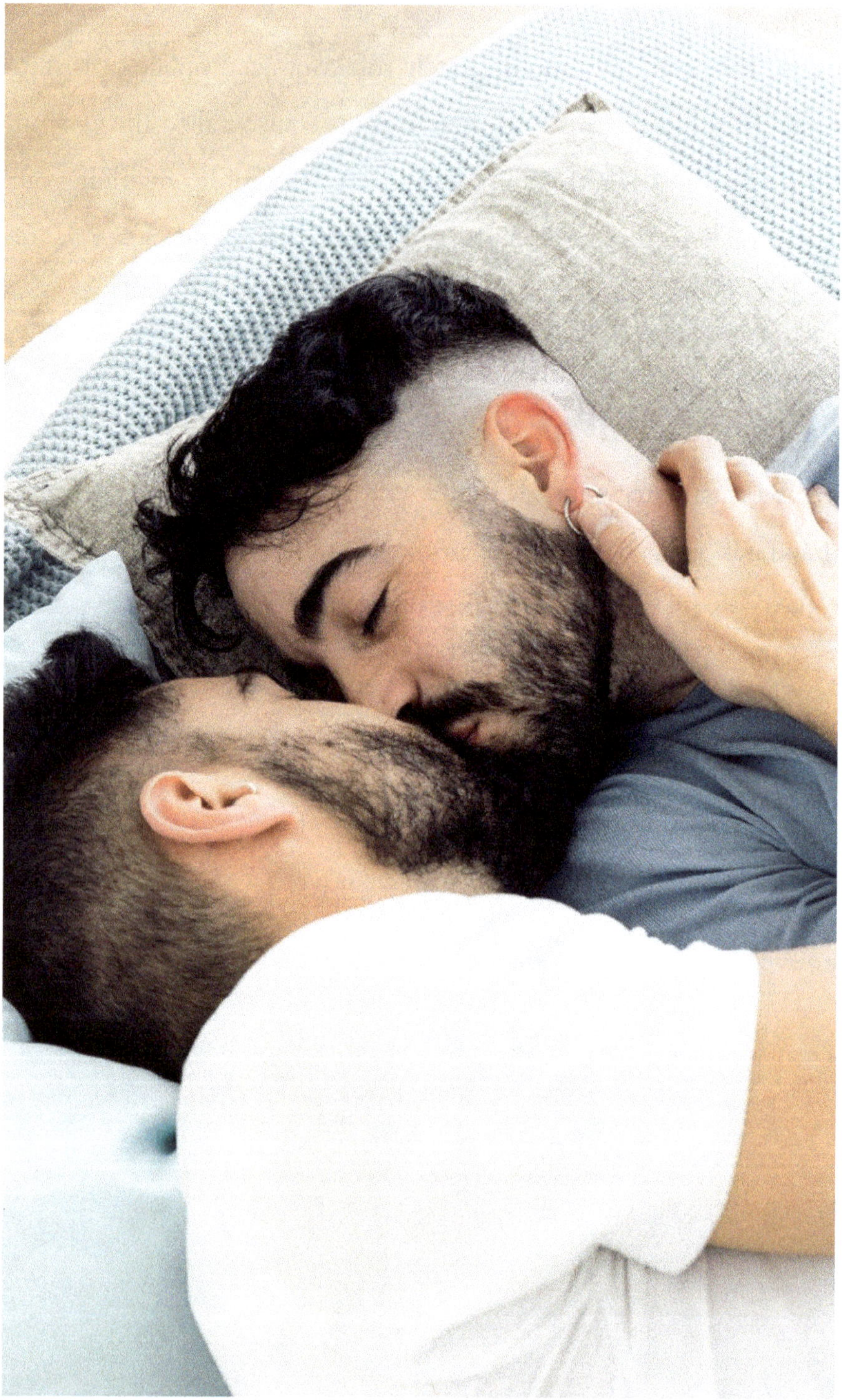

Chapter 7:
Yin and Yang

Everybody perceives the image: the little high contrast half circles that twirl into one another, with a spot of the contrary shading on either side. Just by taking a gander at it, its most fundamental significance is clear: look after equalization. In any case, the importance of Yin and Yang goes a lot further than that.

Foundation

Scarcely any old ways of thinking have been as powerful as Taoism. Created in the fourth century B.C., the way of thinking is revolved around the accomplishment of 'the Way' and discovering agreement and parity inside. At the core of this way of thinking is the image that has come to speak to it as its most identifiable angle: The Yin and Yang.

The image

Considerably more than simply the tattoo on the person from your hand to hand fighting class, the Yin Yang conveys with it a profound implying that is as basic as it is significant.

To get it, how about we separate the image into its two constituent parts. The Yin, or the clouded side, is related with everything hard, negative, cool, wet, and ladylike. The Yang, or the light side, is related to things delicate, positive, warm, dry, and manly.

In any case, in spite of the brutal juxtaposition of their appearances, Yin and Yang are not direct inverses. Truth be told, it is significant that each side has a smidgen of the other in it. That is the way you end up with a wave's peak being Yang and its trough being Yin.

Yin and Yang in regular day to day existence

Actually, Yin and Yang are in all things, and most things are a smidgen of both. An eggshell is Yang; however, the egg inside is Yin.

Wheat in the field is Yang, yet once it is collected, it moves toward becoming Yin. One can transform into the other, and the best things in life lie at the juncture of the two.

The idea of Yin and Yang is at the core of Chinese drug. Have you at any point pondered, for instance, why Chinese individuals drink so much boiling water? It is tied in with offsetting the body's Yin and Yang. It couldn't be any more obvious; the equalization of the two is the most significant angle. The two powers are restricting, however integral.

Nourishment

Chinese nourishment, likewise, is fragmented without a comprehension of Yin and Yang. Yang sustenance's are those who are fiery or sweet. Like the glow that Yang instills, Yang sustenance's are frequently those in warm hues like red and orange.

Yin sustenance's are those who are salty or harsh. They are cool in shading and are regularly developed in water. Models incorporate tofu and soy sauce.

Everybody realizes plain tofu is not the most tantalizing dish. In any case, pair it with some bean stew peppers, a la the Mapo style, and it is the most loved in Chinese cafés around the world.

Despite the fact that all in all, a few dishes are more one than different, components of both Yin and Yang ought to be available inside.

The human body

Despite sex, Yin and Yang are both presents in the human body too, and their quality comes and goes with the time. Normally, Yang is more grounded during the day when the sun is out and it is warm.

What's more, Yin takes over during the evening, when its agent, the moon, comes to join the party.

The Impact of Yin and Yang

Furthermore, however Taoism is more a way of thinking than a religion, it instructs that there is a higher power known to man, 'the Way.' Yet as opposed to being all great or all awful, it is a tad bit of both, much the same as Yin and Yang.

So simply like the Taoist idea of Wu Wei, Yin and Yang is about not pushing back, however tolerating life's differences and figuring out how to see the great, and the awful, in all things.

Yin Yang is maybe the most known and reported idea utilized inside Taoism. A beginning definition: Yin/Yang: Two parts that together complete wholeness. Yin and yang are likewise the beginning stage for change.

When something is entire, by definition, it is perpetual and complete. So when you split something into equal parts – yin/yang, it irritates the balance of wholeness. The two parts are pursuing each other as they look for another offset with one another.

The word Yin turns out to signify "obscure side" and Yang "bright side." Yin Yang is the idea of duality framing an entirety. We experience instances of Yin and Yang consistently. As models: night (Yin) and day (Yang), female (Yin) and male (Yang).

More than a large number of years, a lot has been arranged and assembled under different Yin Yang classification frameworks.

The image for Yin Yang is known as the Taijitu. The vast majority simply consider it the yin yang image in the west. The taijitu image has been found in more than one culture and, throughout the years, has come to speak to Taoism.

Essential Concepts Defining the Nature of Yin Yang

Yin Yang is not static. The idea of Yin and Yang streams and changes with time. A straightforward model is contemplating how the day steadily streams into the night. Be that as it may, the length of day and night are evolving.

As the earth ages, its turn is easing back making the length of day and night get longer. Day and night are not static substances. Some of the time, changes in the connection between Yin and Yang can be sensational, where one viewpoint can simply change into the other.

Neither Yin nor Yang is total. Nothing is totally Yin or totally Yang. Every viewpoint contains the starting point for the other angle.

For instance, day moves toward becoming night and after that night moves toward becoming day. Yin and Yang are reliant upon one another with the goal that the meaning of one requires the definition for the other to be finished.

The summation of Yin and Yang structure an entirety. One impact of this is: as one perspective expands different declines to keep up the general equalization of the entirety.

The parity of Yin Yang can be slanted due to outside impacts. Four potential lopsided characteristics exist: abundance in Yin and Yang and lack in Yin and Yang.

These irregular characteristics can be combined: so an abundance of Yin can likewise recreate a Yang lack and the other way around.

For instance, this idea is particularly significant for Chinese mending rehearses. So an abundance of Yang brings about a fever. An overabundance of Yin could mean the amassing of liquids in the body. Chinese mending looks at an individual's wellbeing by utilizing the eight standards: Internal and External improvements, Deficiency and Excesses, Cold and Heat and Yin and Yang.

Yin Yang can be subdivided into extra Yin and Yang viewpoints. For instance, a Yang part of Heat: can be additionally subdivided into a Yin warm or Yang consuming.

Extra rules that characterize Yin and Yang characteristics exist. The ideas recorded here are only a beginning stage to delineate the idea of Yin and Yang.

For the most part, as a training, Taoism works superbly of not codifying life. Incidentally, this wasn't valid about yin Yang, since over history many Taoist's have attempted to codify what is Yin and what is Yang. Commonly Taoist writings will list a couple of instances of Yin and Yang and afterward wander off to the following point.

For instance, return to the Taoist entry cited above from the Tao Te Ching. You will find a couple of extra angles to Yin and Yang; however, the perusing is certainly not a total definition either. The writer of this section completely anticipates that you, as the peruser, should go out and to investigate the thoughts all alone.

You can endlessly dive into Yin Yang because of its relative nature.

Extra material for Yin Yang can be perused here:

The Flow of Yin and Yang

Presently overlook all that you have found out about Yin and Yang for a minute. A more clear comprehension of Yin Yang requires thinking once more into the Tao. The Tao can be considered as the crucial outright. Upon assessment: the nature of the Tao extends out.

This procedure of extension characterizes an example, parting separated into better and better designs. Yin and Yang are where recognition demarks the Tao's venture into one and afterward one into two.

Taoism, as a training, appreciates inspecting designs. Throughout the years, incalculable organizations of Taoism have framed and a considerable amount of writing composed over the depiction and portrayal of these examples.

Frequently Taoists utilize the idea of Yin Yang as a natural beginning layout to work with examples.

For instance, Qigong depends on the examples of breath and physical development. Information of real examples frames the premise of this Taoist practice to keep a body sound.

The human body and its developments are separated by Yin and Yang classifications. So the chest area compares to the Yang, while the lower body roots into the Yin. The body's middle is the place the Yin and Yang meet. Qi Gong activities are assembled and clarified as far as Yin and Yang to help classify the body's harmonies into a working practice.

The information of Yin or Yang is not required to perform Qi Gong. Rather, it is an extra channel which causes individuals interface with the training.

Another model is Taoist divination inside the Book of Changes/I Ching. Divination in Taoism is a routine with regards to looking at human communications dependent on surely understood mental examples.

To create an outcome either coins or yarrow stalks are hurled down to shape an example. The examples produced compare to Yin and Yang characterized characteristics.

The idea of the Yin and Yang example is connected to the brain research existing apart from everything else to return guidance for the individual posing the inquiry.

Yin Yang is a key part of the Taoist idea. We in every case, normally apply human-based qualities over normally happening examples. Be that as it may, recall it is likewise significant not to pursue better and better portrayals of these examples, to do so is pursue down interminability.

Yin Yang is an arrangement of perceiving how to separate out examples in our life while additionally unwinding to acknowledge the general entire and complete nature of the Tao.

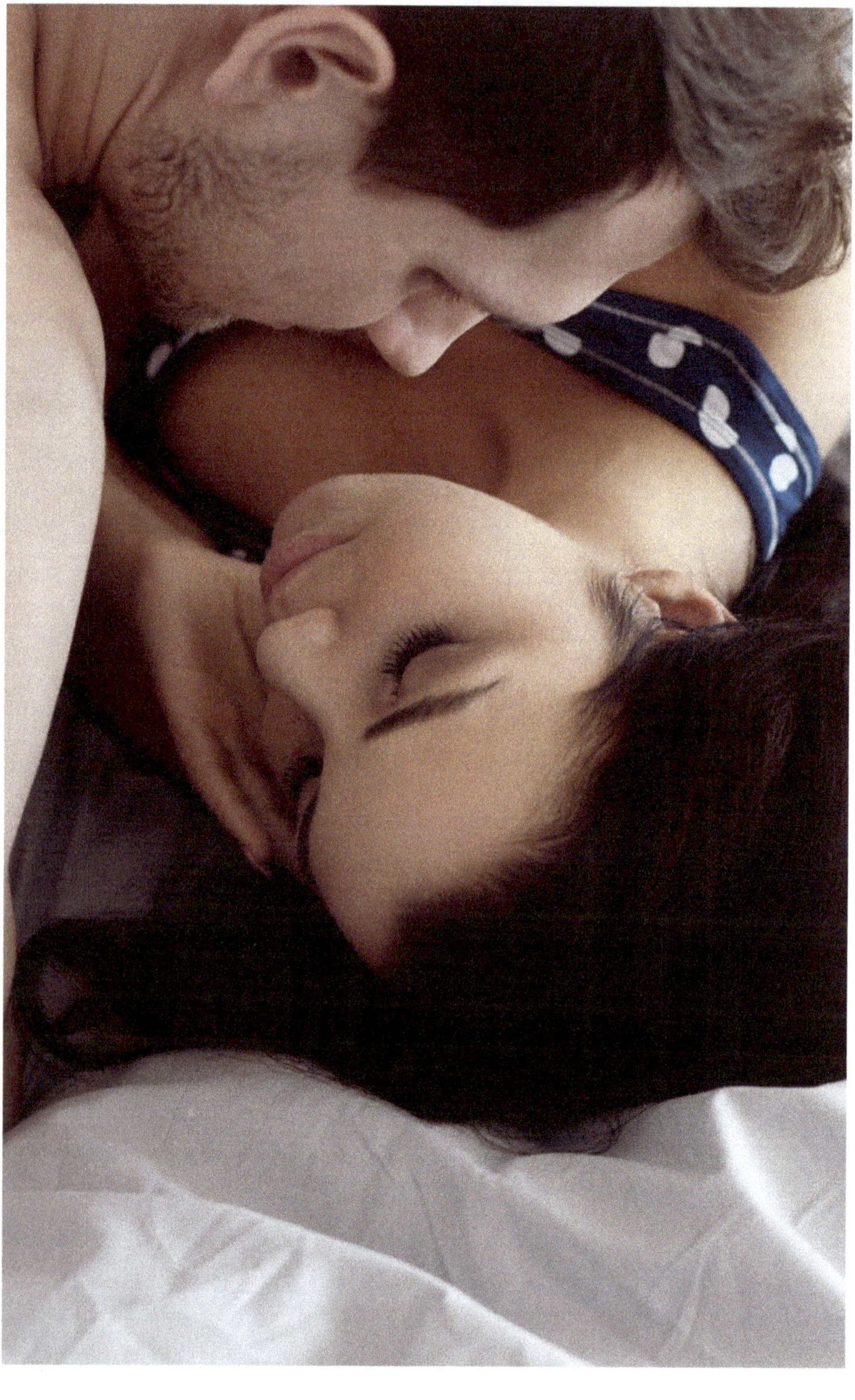

Chapter 8: Shiva and Shakti

Among the characteristics of the Chakras we meet two significant images: Shiva and Shakti.

- SHIVA symbolizes awareness, the manly guideline.
- SHAKTI symbolizes the female guideline, the initiating force and vitality.

At whatever point a power winds up dynamic, and any place vitality exists, Shakti is working. Different expressions for these basic standards are Purusha and Prakriti; Purusha is cognizance and Prakriti is nature.

Ruler Shiva is commonly depicted holding a trident, which speaks to the trinity of Īshwara, Purusha and Prakriti.

Īshwara is the inescapable, unceasing, shapeless celestial rule; Purusha is the Ātmā and Prakriti is the manifestation, nature. An electric light can be utilized to clarify their relationship.

The electric flow, which is the wellspring of the light, is Īshwara; the light is Purusha, and the item that is lit up is Prakriti.

Shakti (or Prakriti) implies vitality, control, development, change, nature. It is the maternal guideline — the supplier, plenitude. In the human, just as in the set of all animals, the mother offers sustenance, warmth and security.

There is no more prominent love than the affection for a mother. The mother conveys and supports the youngster in her own body. When it is conceived, she furnishes it with mother's milk and raises it at the sacrifice of her own self until it ends up independent.

Shiva (or Purusha), then again, is unadulterated awareness – the perpetual, boundless and unswayable onlooker. Purusha has no wanted at all; these are intrinsic just in Prakriti. Purusha is the vacant, clear screen onto which Prakriti ventures her beautiful film.

Shiva and Shakti are manifestations of the across the divine board awareness - different sides of a similar coin. In numerous photos, these two base forces are each delineated as being one portion of a similar picture; one side female and one side male.

The left side is the Divine Mother, Pārvatī, the "ladylike" vitality, and the correct side speaks to Shiva, the "manly" awareness.

Through the parting of the primordial standard at the coming of creation, the duality inside our lives appeared, together with a solid power that is always endeavoring to re-join with the other part.

Just when Shiva and Shakti consolidate can activity, development and creation emerge. Until vitality is impregnated with cognizance, it is oblivious, confused, erratic and "dazzle." Vitality alone can create nothing; awareness presents to its substance, structure and bearing.

Then again, cognizance without vitality is dormant power, dozing vitality, and all alone cannot be the reason for anything. Similarly, as Prakriti without Purusha cannot act, and the other way around, Purusha without Prakriti is additionally unequipped for making anything.

The significance of Shiva and Shakti is once in a while misconstrued when Shiva and Shakti are viewed as "man" and "lady," and their association is viewed as a sexual relationship.

Sexuality is something totally common, and misconception emerges just when sexuality and otherworldliness are blended.

- Sexuality is the association between man and lady.
- Otherworldliness is the association of the human and the perfect cognizance.

Shiva and Shakti exist inside every one of us as the manly and female standards. This affects the physical level – it is the reason for sexual fascination. Inside man, there exists an inclination towards the ladylike characteristics, and inside lady a propensity towards the manly.

Through this, the manly awareness is pulled in by the ladylike and the other way around. If both are in parity there is no sexual fascination; however, if a propensity for the manly prevails in man, or the ladylike in lady, these outcomes in an inclination for a homosexual accomplice.

Shiva dwells in the Sahasrāra Chakra and Shakti in the Mūlādhāra Chakra. Whenever Prakriti and Purusha join in the Sahasrāra Chakra, learning, knower and the object of information become one.

When we have encountered, this no wants to stay inside us since we understand unequivocally that all that we have ever longed for is conveyed inside us. In this condition of total cognizance, there are no polarities and subsequently no more distresses; there is just everlasting bliss, unrestricted love, boundless empathy, and all-out comprehension for every living being.

For whatever length of time that cognizance is associated with the physical body it cannot remain continually in the Sahasrāra Chakra thus comes back to the living arrangement of the Ātmā in the Heart Center (Anāhata Chakra).

An acknowledged individual consistently thinks, feels and acts from the heart. Inserted in everlasting affection and interminable joy, that individual is constantly aware of the undying Ātmā, the sea of joy, and their awareness is always associated with the heavenly cognizance.

- Shakti is the nurturing affection for God that encompasses us with warmth, mindful and assurance.
- Shiva is the fatherly love of God that gives us cognizance, lucidity and learning.

I wish for you the gift of the Divine Mother who lives inside you as vitality and imperativeness, and the gift of the Divine Father who dwells inside you as cognizance and information.

May they generally deal with you, secure you and guide you, and in their limitless love lead you to the infinite cognizance.

As per Shaivism, one of the real parts of yogic way of thinking, there is a perfect manly vitality that appears as the Hindu god, Shiva, and an awesome ladylike vitality that appears as the goddess, Shakti. Both Shiva and Shakti are alive in the two people.

We all have divine manly (Shiva) viewpoints and perfect female (Shakti) perspectives to our being. It is said that our female side dwells on our left side while the manly lives on our correct side.

We hold these energies inside us and, when joined together, there is a finished parity, satisfaction and nearness inside our very being. Getting to every one of our celestial natures — both manly and ladylike — can be both edifying and astounding. Be that as it may, we have to recollect that we convey inside us the two parts of the Divine. Here we'll become acquainted with increasingly about the characteristics of Shiva vitality just as Shakti vitality, at that point, at long last, the nature of these awesome energies joined.

The Nature of Shakti Energy

Shakti is wonderfully beautiful with a streaming and shape-shifting quality to her — holding onto reality as a move. She is liquid, streaming and capably adaptable.

Shakti vitality can be fiercely exotic, crude and expressive. Shakti vitality can be seen in everything that lives as the manifest, while Shiva vitality is nebulous.

Things that have just appeared are made of Shakti vitality. These two supernaturally sacrosanct energies are equivalent and inverse powers. We cannot have one without the other.

We can coordinate Shiva and Shakti inside our inward awareness, inside our whole existence. These hallowed forces can open us up and change our very being.

The Shakti vitality inside us can appear as prana, that life power vitality that courses through our Nadis, or unobtrusive vitality channels. It can likewise appear as kundalini vitality, that wound vitality that untruths torpid at the base of the spine until it is released.

At the point when this occurs, a kundalini arousing happens, in which the Shakti vitality stirs and travels through the focal channel, or the Sushumna Nadi, along which the seven chakras dwell. This is when profound purifying, recuperating and change happens — and everything occurs through the development of Shakti vitality inside.

We can feel our Shiva vitality when we are the observer of the Shakti. When we sit in reflection, developing clear nearness and reason, we are resting inside our internal Shiva nature.

Shiva holds space for Shakti to travel through. Shiva provides guidance to Shakti's shape-shifting fiery stream.

The Nature of Shiva Energy

Shiva is another name for the Absolute Reality or Absolute Consciousness that makes up our universe.

Shiva is the otherworldly part of enormous awareness or the Source of everything and all that is. Shiva, in the entirety of his resolute joining between the interior world and the outside world, is regularly known as the Lord of Yoga. The intensity of Shiva's awareness can bring incredible internal quality and extensive size.

In the custom of Shaivism, Shiva is perpetually in association with Shakti, his supernaturally ladylike partner. The idea of Shiva vitality is unfaltering, steady, quiet, solid and absolutely unaffected with complete nearness.

Shiva speaks to the condition of being unaffected by agony or enduring expedited by the outside world. He is focused, grounded and sympathetic. We can summon his unadulterated nearness through contemplation to bring in the phenomenal characteristics of Shiva into our very own being.

Heading, reason, opportunity, and mindfulness — these are our supernaturally manly characteristics. The manly vitality of Shiva knows about everything that comes into creation.

Every one of the things of creation are birthed through the ladylike part of Shakti, and we all include these characteristics inside us also. They are move, development, power, vitality, and the opportunity to turn into.

Shiva is unadulterated being in its stillness. Shakti is unadulterated, getting to be in the entirety of her stream and imagination just as her unending opening to plausibility.

Your internal manly side knows what his identity is and is intentional in his knowing. There is profound shrewdness and limit with regards to mindfulness inside Shiva.

Shiva-Shakti Union

In association, Shiva and Shakti make up the half-lady master known as Ardhanarishvara.

The picture of Shiva-Shakti in associate is a really beautiful one to look at. This male/female figure demonstrates the association of manly and ladylike parts of our being, which realizes an otherworldly wholeness inside.

Shiva is the yogi god with his exposed middle and built legs, with dreadlocks and a snake around his neck. He conveys a trident and has a quiet face. Shakti has long hair, huge almond molded eyes and fragile highlights.

She wears a streaming silk fabric and one of her feet is brought up in a move. The picture passes on complete parity, satisfaction, and nearness. This is Shiva-Shakti — the association of hallowed manly and female cognizance that exists in us and all through the Cosmos.

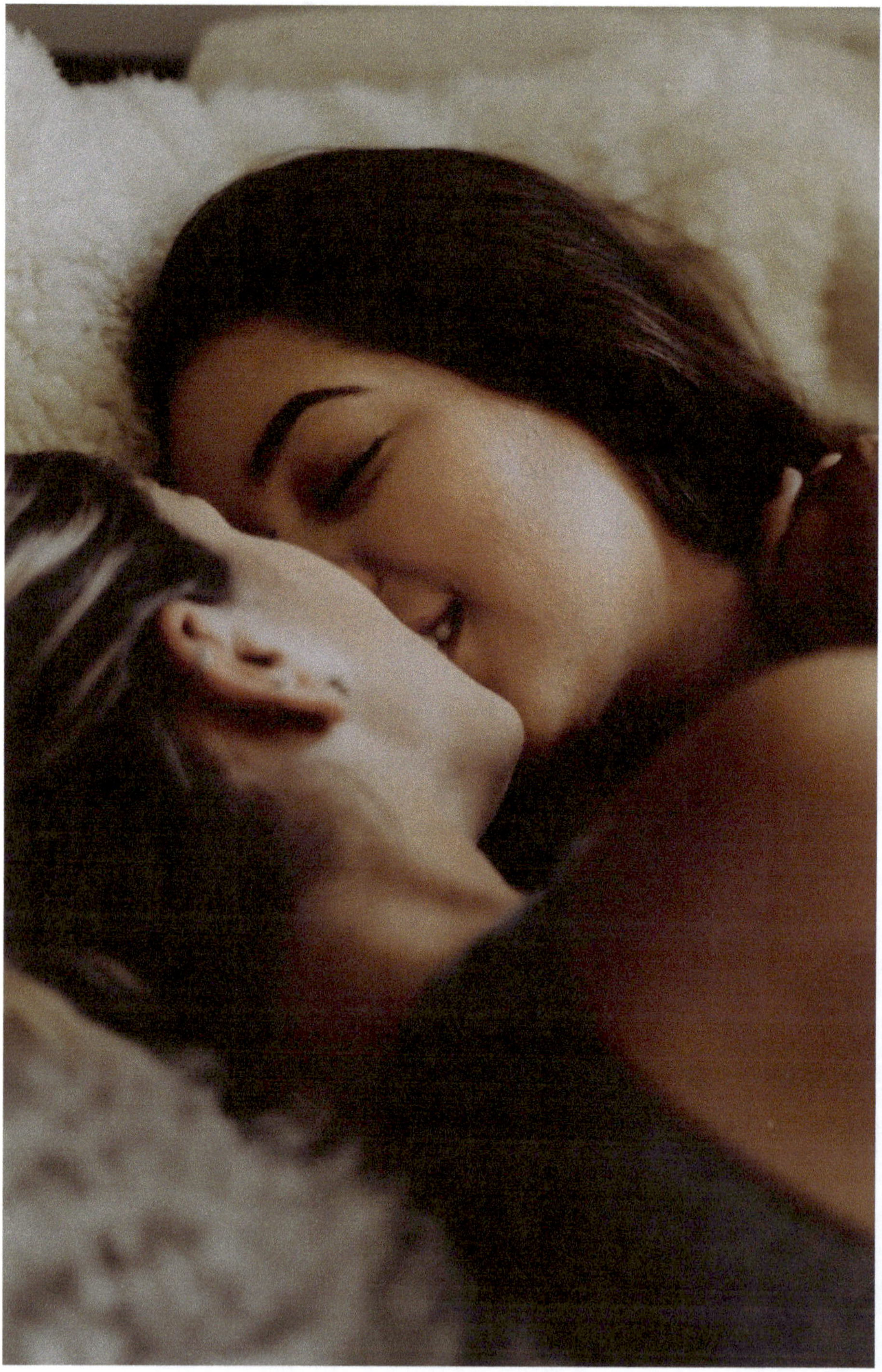

Conclusion

Too often, we become absorbed in work, family life, and home our never-ending list of obligations and we forget that life is supposed to be enjoyed.

We rarely hold pleasure up as one of the main goals in life, and it is time that we change our mindsets and embrace the fact that life has much more to offer us. No longer do you need to drudge through each day, only to wake up and begin the routine all over again.

Instead, let this book be a lesson to you that pleasure is equally as important as a duty, and to truly have a balanced life you must indulge in both.

Whether sexual or non-sexual, romantic, or non-romantic, there is so much pleasure within our world that we deprive ourselves of, or simply don't even know exists.

The Kama Sutra reminds us to slow down and allow ourselves the freedom to explore our innermost wants and desires, so that we may see the true beauty in life. The Kama Sutra is spiritual in nature, and it doesn't matter if you believe in a religion or not, you too should be able to see the profoundness that is contained within.

Allowing yourself to reach a higher plane of fulfillment is indescribable, and thankfully this book can help guide you to that place.

So, take a moment, close your eyes, and think about everything that makes you feel alive. Now, give yourself the freedom to partake in all of those pleasures, and then you will truly understand the power of the Kama Sutra.

Finally, if you found this book useful in any way, a review on Amazon is always appreciated!

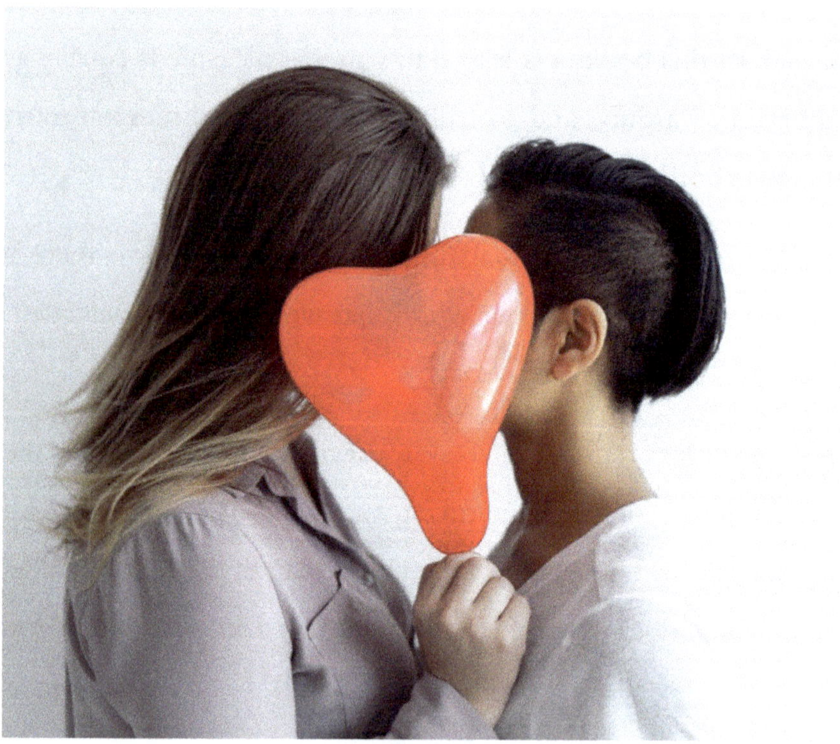

CPSIA information can be obtained
at www.ICGtesting.com
Printed in the USA
LVHW081740280621
691285LV00027B/314

9 781802 662634